Carb Cycling for Beginners

Carb Cycling for Beginners

Simple Recipes and Exercises for Weight Loss, Reactivating Metabolism and Muscle Building

Tiffany Nicholas

Dedication

This diet plan book is dedicated to **You!**

You that want to lose weight but want to maintain your lifestyle.

TERMS & CONDITIONS

All Rights Reserved

No part of this cookbook may be reproduced or transmitted in any form whatsoever, electronics mechanical, including photocopying, or by any informational storage or retrieval system without expressed written, dated and signal permission from the author.

Copyright © by Tiffany Nicholas (2020)

Disclaimer

The information in this book should not be used for diagnosing or treating any health problem. Not all diet and exercise plans suit everyone. You should always consult a trained medical professional before starting a diet, taking any form of medication, or embarking on any fitness or weight-training program. The author and publisher disclaim any liability arising directly or indirectly from the use of this book.

Always follow safety and commonsense cooking protocol while using kitchen utensils, operating ovens and stoves, and handling uncooked food. If children are assisting in the preparation of any recipe, they should always be supervised by an adult. Readers are encouraged to seek professional help when is required.

This guide is for informational purposes only and the author does not accept any responsibilities for any liabilities resulting from the use of this information. While every attempt has been made to verify the information provided here, the author cannot assume any responsibility for errors, inaccuracies or omission.

Simple Recipes and Exercises for Rapid Weight Loss, Increased Energy and Enhanced Health.

TABLE OF CONTENTS

TABLE OF CONTENTS	7
INTRODUCTION	1
WHY CARB CYCLING	5
FUNDAMENTALS OF CARB CYCLING	11
GETTING STARTED	24
CARB CYCLING DIET PLAN	59
LOW CARB DAYS RECIPES	71
HIGH CARB DAYS RECIPES	76
CONCLUSION	81

INTRODUCTION

There are many information and many diets out there either online or offline when it comes to weight management. What we discovered was that many of these diets don't address the underlying factors that make the management of weight easier, such as perception, self-image, and the skills to maintaining the weight loss processes.

The above attributes are the foundation of our behavior and are known to be the primary sources of determinants when it comes to what we will experience in our lives. These determinants include weight management and any other behavioral issues. Those issues include thoughts, feelings and actions. So many times that we have the impression that the problems are symptoms but failed to check the underlying factors that happen to be the primary issues.

Dealing with the factors mentioned above will bring out advantages that are long terms, especially in situations such as for overweight and weight problems. A symptom such as overweight will only be taken care if there are fundamental guidelines that not only come with the diet plan but are psychological.

How do you handle a diet plan that stipulates that you are to religiously follow specific rules that can't be cheated or ignore! The main reason why most of the diet plans failed is that it does not put into consideration the real nature of human beings.

Now let's dive into the psychological aspect of weight management. You will be having low self-image if you accept that you are overweight and obese when no figure supports it. The message you are sending to your inner being is that you are worthless, and don't have what it takes to be useful to yourself, and society.

Remember that overweight is BMI of 25.0 to 29.9 kg/m2, while a healthy BMI is between 18.5 to 24.9 kg/m2. Having a number lower is considered as being underweight. To be known as obese, your BMI must be 30.0 kg/m2 or higher. But BMI of 40.0 kg/m2 is known as morbid obesity. So you are expected to know and understanding these numbers before you castigate yourself or subject yourself to mental slavery.

Once this has been taken care of, this book contains proven diet that will help you in fixing meals that will change your lifestyle without having to be strict about the change of lifestyle. Ordinarily, we all want to leave a free life!

I'm introducing to you a diet plan that I have observed over some years and can categorically tell you that this is a way to lose weight fast without going crazy with hunger and deprivation-Carb Cycling diet.

Carb cycling is a form of a diet plan that allows you to mix higher carbohydrates days with low carbohydrates days and you may decide to change some days to either moderate carb days or no-carb days to burn fat and supercharge weight loss.

Carb cycling diet does not make me suffer some form of negative consequences of a simple low carb diet plan that may deprive my body of macronutrients. I have discovered that the majority of the diet programs in the markets usually limit food choices. Still, carb cycling activates several general healthy eating guidelines and consuming a higher amount of carbs in some days. This diet plan will force the body to metabolize fat and protein so to generate a substance known as ketone.

With carb cycling, you can decide to make three days out of the seven days in a week to be of low carb followed by another three days to high carb days and make the last one day to be either no or moderate carb day. And it can be alternated. In plain language, the calorie intake during the low carb day should be low, while calorie intake during the high carb days should be higher.

It is advised first to calculate your required daily calorie intake and work out the needed quantity of carb to be consumed.

This book will expose all the necessary methods, tools, shopping list, what to avoid, workouts to add with carb cycling and the recipes that will make your journey in losing fat more accessible.

Chapter 1

WHY CARB CYCLING

It is fantastic when guarded nutritional concepts meant for the elite athletes and professional bodybuilders are now open secrets! Secrets such as macros counts, eating for the recomposition of body, and re-feeding days. You may not necessarily need to make use of all of these secrets, but if you are targeting a specific fitness goal, they will readily become your arsenal.

There have been several diets that trend and go into waves. Some of these diets made us afraid of eating too much fat, thereby making us run away from carbs. Our fear of running away from carbs, as suggested by all of these diets are justified, as carbs make a large portion of our daily calories. So consuming too much of carb is not too good, and lead to problems, especially when looking for ways to lose weight or getting healthier.

So choosing to cut out entirely carbs won't be necessary as

there is a diet that teaches how to eat the right kinds of carbs such as brown rice and oats that will not only give your body fuel to handle the exercises but also able to carry out the daily routines. No wonder some people have opted for another nutritional strategy known as carb cycling. Carb cycling is a way to alternate between low carb days and high carb days. The following are why and what you need to know about carb cycling—not forgetting to tell if carb cycling diet is appropriate for you.

WHAT IS CARB CYCLING?

Carb cycling is a way to eat a higher amount of carbs one day, and then the next day to eat a lower amount of carbs. Alternate the arrangement between these two options throughout the week. Alternating the arrangement will largely depend on the type of activities you engage during each day. What you want to achieve is to have high carbs during the day you participate in high activities and low carbs when you are less active.

When you go on work out your body will make use of a large number of carbs, that's the reason why you need more during the exercise days. As you will burn more calories during the workout than during the day, you have lesser daily routines.

WHO IS CARB CYCLING FOR?

Studies showed that there are two main groups of people that carb cycling is appropriate for- endurance athletes and people that are very active but are on low carb diets.

Professional endurance athletes that engage in sports such as soccer, swimming, cycling, and running, have been discovered to reducing their consumption of carbs before entering into the primary season as it will help their body in better-utilizing carbs.

For those that are interested in the management of their weights or fat loss, carb cycling is a great way to achieve it. The general notion is that eating lower carb diet such as keto will help in weight control and enjoying optimal health. It is no secret that carbohydrates are the primary fuel for working muscles when in a high-intensity workout. So eating carbs before and after high-intensive activities is needed so to get along.

DIFFERENCE BETWEEN LOW CARB DAYS AND KETO

Carb cycling is known to be popular with those who follow keto diet- low-carbs, high-fat. However, you don't need to be consuming a high-fat diet to have the benefits of carb cycling. As you can manipulate any diet to cycle your carbs. It will even be better not to carb cycle while on keto, especially when you are new to the diet. As the general rule of the ketogenic diet is to make sure that the carbs are low and the fat is so high that ketones are fueling the body.

Don't forget that the main reason for following a ketogenic diet is to make use of fat as fuel instead of carb, so taking body in and out of ketosis will defeat the purpose and may lead to thinking that the eating style is not working.

Another angle to look at it is that low carb does not have clear definitions as most guidelines suggest to make it around 150 grams daily when compared to keto that is around 50 gram daily.

THINGS TO KNOW BEFORE JOINING CARB CYCLING

To start carb cycling, there are some basic things that you have to know, and are;

Amount of calories needed

You have to establish the daily calorie goal aimed for all days.

The general rule:

To lose weight: You have to multiply bodyweight by 10 (This will give the calorie needed for each day).

For weight maintenance: You have to multiply bodyweight by 12.

For weight gain: You have to multiply bodyweight by 15.

Balance the Macros

• Divide the calories among the main macronutrients such as fats, carbs, and fat.

• Carbs and protein provide four calories per gram.

• Fat provides nine calories per gram.

- It is advised to aim for 1 gm of protein per pound of body weight and make up the rest of the calorie with good fats.

Avoid mixing the fiber

Whenever you have planned to eat lesser carbohydrates, it is advised to keep the fiber. Engaging in low carb days are no excuse for you to dump your fruits. Your focus should be on how to remove added sugar and other refined carbs such as bagels and muffins from your food. Add fruits that are fiber and nutrient-rich vegetables, fruits and quality grains.

Eat enough food, even while on low-carb days.

Note that brains run on the carb, especially sugar glucose. So it implies that whenever there is no carb, the body will make use of other sources such as protein, which is not good when you are looking for ways to build lean muscle. This is the reasons why it is essential to consume more than 130 gm of carbs during the low-carb days.

Chapter 2

FUNDAMENTALS OF CARB CYCLING

Now to start the journey!

As you are about to start the journey to weight loss, it is advisable to have detailed proactive plan that will make the trip easy, organize, and eventful.

There are five smart fundamentals to follow in this journey if you want to have optimal results. This chapter will illustrate and explain how to achieve this feat.

FIVE FUNDAMENTALS TO CARB CYCLING

1. Your goal to weight loss must be specific:

You must have a specific purpose like "My goal is to lose 50 pounds," or "My goal is to have six-packs," or "My goal is to reduce blood pressure to 120/180," Don't generalize your goal by "I want to lose weight," or "I want to reduce my blood pressure," or "I want to look healthy". They are ordinary goals and not a specific type of goal that will drive you to be detailed about what to do to achieve the goal.

Know that every journey that has a beginning and must surely has an end. So if you are vague or generalize about a goal, what you are trying to do is given the unspecific goal time, or be left uncompleted when it proves difficult to be accomplished. With this type of mindset of having a specific goal, you will build the right character in achieving your goal. And you may hate yourself for never drive your inner being to make what you want. Your goal is to tell your inner self what you want to achieve individually, and it must be completed.

Assignment:

My goal is to.......

2. Your plan must be measurable:

Your plan must be measurable to make the goal achievable. Never you based your progress on what people are telling you about yourself, or looking in the mirror and conclude that you have achieved the goal. Let your weight-loss and health goal be precise and detailed in either of the following;

Assignment 1:

My desired weight in...kg/....pounds

My desired measurement in ...inches/ ....centimeters

My Thigh...

My Waist...

My Hips.....

My Neck.....

My Chest.....

My blood pressure......

My Glucose tolerance......

My Blood panel........

Etc.

Assignment 2:

In this section, you will have to take measurement of your body now before you embark on the carb cycling journey. This initial measurement will be your bases to achieve your goal. The differences in the numbers when you have shed some weight will be the indicators to tell you that you are on the right track. So it is advisable to keep this record in a safe place.

Date:

Weight:

Clothing Sizes:

Neck in ....inches (take the measurement of the circumference of your neck)

Chest in.... inches (take the measurement of the circumference of your chest, keeping the arms at your side)

Waist in.... inches (take the measurement at the navel)

Hips in.... inches (take the measurement at the widest point, that's 6 to 8 inches below the waist)

Thigh in..... inches (take the measurement of the right thigh at about 8 inches above the knee)

Note: Keep this information in a safe place for before and after comparisons.

3. Your goal must be attainable:

Your goal must be what you can do within your reach. Meaning if your goal requires four hours of time and activities a day, and you are a single mother that's on a full-time job. This is not attainable as the goal is not realistic. Instead, it is better to set 1 hour that you can easily attain with your daily scheduled activities. Another type of situation is if your goal requires a piece of expensive equipment and you can't afford it, it is better to reconsider the goal. So it is better to set goals that are attainable and can fit your present situation.

Assignment:

What are the things that will make my goal attainable?

4. Your goal must be realistic:

The truth of this journey is that it must be realistic. Imagine having a goal of losing 250 pounds within three months! And quite alright, you know you cannot achieve this feat. I can assure you that disappointment will be your sorry case. Don't forget that disappointment will put your journey into jeopardy, and it will give your emotion the opportunity to withdraw from the journey.

If your goal is to lose 250 pounds, it is advised to give yourself time to be able to achieve it. Let it be something like, "I will lose 250 pounds by ...date, two and half years from now". So it is not having a goal of losing 250 pounds within three months. Instead, it is possible to lose 30 pounds within three months.

Remember that attainable goal and realistic goal go hand in hand. So you are expected to set goals that you know you can achieve physically and attainable. Your goals should be able to fit into your lifestyle.

To know the estimation of the amount of weight you can reasonably lose weekly is for you to take your current weight, divide it by 100. The answer is the approximation of the amount of weight that you can lose safely weekly. For instance, a person that weighs 190 pounds, to know the amount that can be easily lost is to divide 190 by 100. So the answer is 1.9 pounds. However, this is a rough estimate.

Assignment:

What are the things that will make my goal realistic?

5. Your goal must be sensitive:

To set a goal that is important to your health and happiness, the goal must be sensitive. For this goal to be achieved, there must not be room for procrastination and lapses. You should never allow room for excuses, and there must be a realistic deadline. Set a clear time frame for your goal to be achieved.

Assignment:

I must reach my goal by...... (Date)

STOCK UP

Do you realize that if you stock up your kitchen with all things that will encourage you in your journey to carb cycling goals, it will drive you in achieving your short and long term success? So if you want to realize your desired goal quickly, it is advised to surround yourself with what will encourage you in keeping up with your set goals?

So whenever you go to the grocery store, it is expected of you always to buy things that will support your journey in carb cycling. You have to keep reminding yourself that to achieve your goal to be fit and healthy is more important than satisfying your cravings for things that won't support your goals.

It is recommended that you do anything that will always help in keeping your fitness desire high and low your temptations when you get to the grocery store until buying what matters becomes your habit.

GET RID OF UNWANTED FOODS

After you have getting foods and things to help you in your journey to carb cycling, you will need to store them. So it is advisable to throw out or give out the foods in your house that may distract you from achieving your goals. It doesn't matter whether you have enough room to stock them; it is better to donate or throw them out to avoid distraction.

The following are the foods to be removed from your store or kitchen:

Hard alcohol

Cookies

Fried foods

Wine

Chocolate

Frozen meals

Chips

Ice cream

Candy

White and wheat bread

Soda

Baked goods

Crackers

Juice

Beer

Also, get rid of the foods that contain these ingredients:

White flour

Brown sugar

Raw sugar

Hydrogenated oils

White sugar

Corn syrup

Maple syrup

Honey

White rice

Remember that it is better to clean out your house of junk so to do yourself a huge favor. Doing this is like giving yourself support by making your environment ready for your journey.

HOW TO COMBINE YOUR FOODS FOR OPTIMAL RESULTS

The way you combine foods in your meals is critical as it will encourage you in your journey of weight loss.

HOW TO COMBINE FOODS ON HIGH-CARB DAYS

On these days you are expected to select one protein and one carbohydrate for every meal you will be preparing, provided you want fast results. Don't forget that protein is the building block that will help in the growing and maintenance of muscles, while carbohydrates are the fuel that will feed your metabolism. According to the guidelines on carb cycling, fats are not to be combined on high-carb days to avoid getting extra calorie. It is recommended that you add vegetables to every meal as they are a source of minerals, vitamins, and fiber, but not compulsory during the high-carb days. You don't need to eat veggies during the high-carb day when you are full.

HOW TO COMBINE FOODS ON LOW-CARB DAYS

Remember that during the low-carb days, protein is compulsory at every meal, with vegetables and fats. It is the function of the protein to prevent the body from cannibalizing your muscle when undergoing rapid fat-loss days. Vegetables provide fiber, minerals, and vitamins, and the fats will help in preventing cravings. Remember that during these days, carbs are not an option, except while on breakfast. I recommend that you eat your breakfast like that of high-carb days, combining with carbs and protein. But don't add carbs to the rest of other meals in the day.

Make sure that you fill your day with vegetable and fats, so to cover for the deficiencies of it during the high-carb days. Though you will be consuming fewer calories on low-carb days, you will discover that you will not be hungry. So you are expected to eat enough protein and vegetables. You may feel sluggish, but remember that your body is burning fat.

HOW TO STOP CRAVINGS FOR FOODS

It's good you have decided to start a transition to a healthier lifestyle. It's natural as no matter how hard you have determined to achieve your goal there would be moments and situations when your body and mind will crave for foods that you have opted not to eat again. Candies, fatty foods, and snacks are delicious and sweet, but they are tough to forgo. Though some of them can be eaten during the cheat days, you must focus on those that will help in promoting health. The following are some of the ways to manage your cravings.

Drink lots of water: Drinking lots of water will bring the sensation of fullness and will help in curbing the urge to eat sweet foods.

Eat high-carb food early: Eat high-fiber foods early in the day as they stay in the stomach, especially small intestine longer, thereby keeping you not hungry.

Consume little good fats: Consume a small amount of good fats not only during the low carb days but every day.

Chew mint: Get favored mint, or breath mint, or toothpaste whenever there is craving. You won't believe how they will suppress your appetite and keep you full.

Chapter 3

GETTING STARTED

WORKOUTS IN CARB CYCLING

We have discovered that the effects of morning exercises are significant and astounding. Starting your day with just 10-minute workout will result in increased energy and productivity during the day. This early workout will bring more sound sleep at night, and lesser sleep since the one done would be sound. Though when starting the exercise, it will be difficult to wake up without the alarm, but within five to six days, your body will be adjusted to wake as at when due.

Regardless of the types of workout, you are doing; you are to warm up before the exercise begins, and relax a bit when you are done. It is not advisable to just start exercise without having to inform your body of what to expect. This warm-up has been known to prevent injury when the exercise begins proper. Another mistake people are making again is not cooling down the body when the exercise stops.

How to warm-up before the real workout

1. March in a place for 45 seconds to one minute.

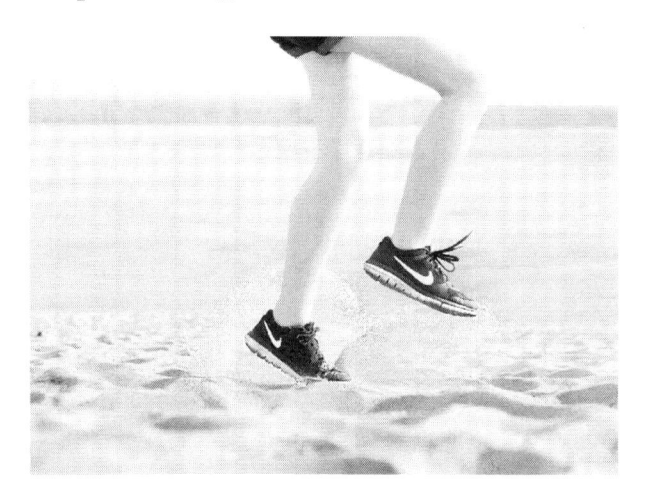

2. Jog in a place for 30-45 seconds.

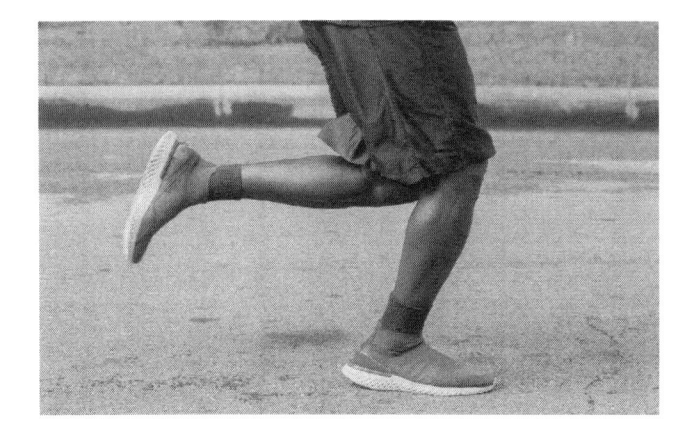

3. And then, finally engage in jumping jack for 30 -45 seconds.

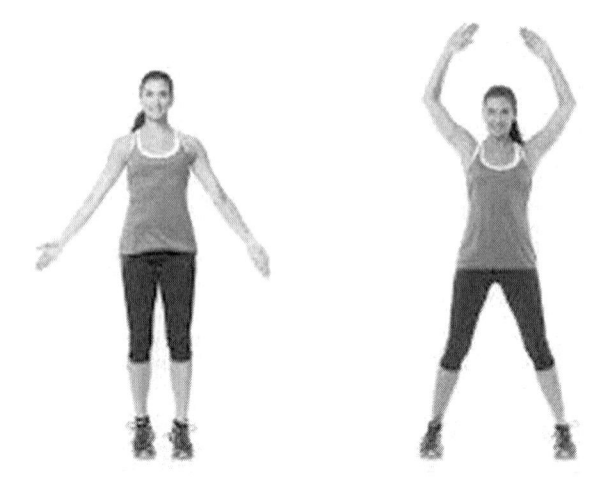

Note: This warm-up should not be more than 5 minutes.

The above three exercises will move your biggest muscle groups, help in increasing the body temperature, and blood flow to the joints and muscles. Warming up has been known to help in contracting and relaxing the muscles faster, thereby making you not having strains and pulls.

WORKOUTS IN CARB CYCLING

1. PLANK

Plank is a form of workout that will work on the core of your body. It will work from the pelvic girdle to the shoulder and the legs. Plank is designed to strengthen the spine, trapezius, rhomboids, and abdominal muscles.

Benefits of the Plank exercise

• Plank exercises are one of the best workouts.

• Planks aids posture.

• Planks can be used to treat back pain.

• Planks help in coordination.

• Planks can be used to improve flexibility.

• Planks are great to enhance metabolism.

• Planks improve mood.

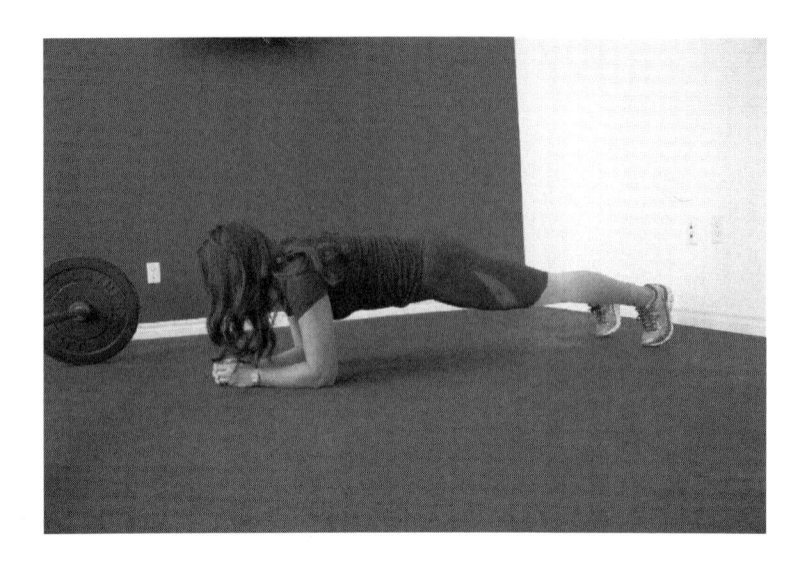

Steps:

1. Lie flat on the stomach with legs flat and upper part of body propping up forearms.

2. Tight lower back and shoulder muscles by raising the hips off the ground.

3. Hold this position between 30 to 45 seconds.

4. Then relax.

Note:

Done five complete of the above processes. Your arms will quivers to shows that it's working.

2. BODYWEIGHT SQUATS

Bodyweight squats are a way of strengthening the lower part of the body. This is done to make significant muscles of the legs functional.

Benefits of Bodyweight squats

• It helps in burning fats and loss of weight.

• This workout can be used to tone the overall body.

• It aids the posture.

• Bodyweight squats can be used to improve flexibility.

• Aids blood circulation.

• It can be used to treat back pain.

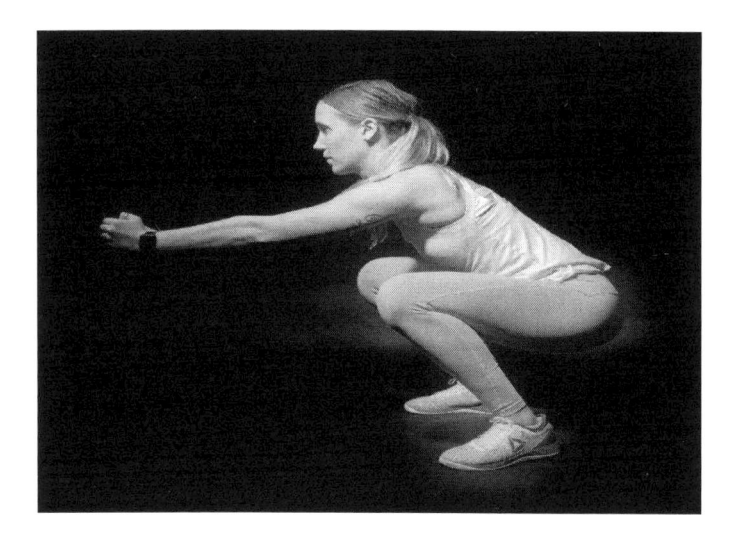

Steps:

1. Stand upright with feet in a position that will look slightly wider than shoulder-width apart.

2. The toes must be pointed straight ahead.

3. Bend the legs and drop buttocks down to the height of knees.

4. The legs should form a 90-degree angle when at the bottom of the movement.

5. Push back upright with weight lean on heels.

6. Squeeze through glutes on the way up.

7. Do the 5 sets of 25 repetitions.

3. WALKING LUNGES

Walking lunges are ways to strengthens lower muscles, and are just modified stationary lunges.

Walking lunges have a significant impact on hips, hamstrings, glutes, calves, abdominals, and quadriceps.

Benefits of Walking lunges

- When the Walking lunges are adequately done, they will help in achieving stable core, as it engages the core and abdominal muscles.

- Walking lunges will aid proper body balance and well coordination.

- It will help in the strengthening of buttocks and legs.

- Walking lunges enhances hip flexibility.

- While some workouts put pressure on the spine, walking lunges helps to reduce the load on the spine.

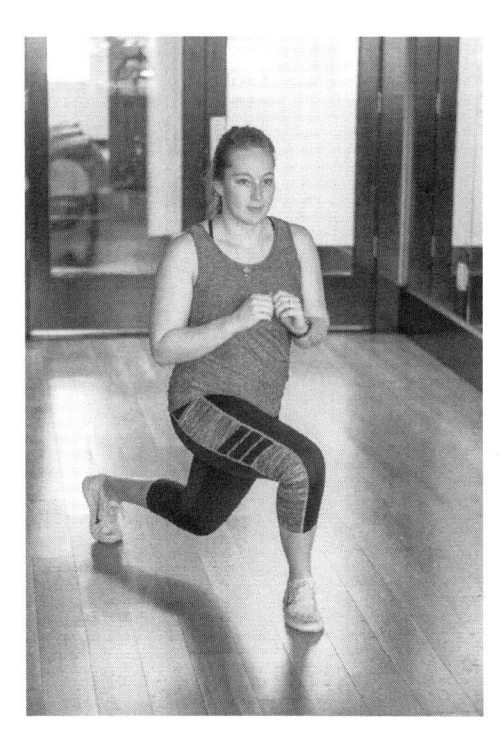

Steps:

1. Stand upright with feet and shoulder-width apart.

2. Take a large step forward with the right leg.

3. Drop the body down for the back leg to touch the ground.

4. Push down the front heel and stand back upright.

5. Repeat the steps with the left leg.

6. Do 5 sets of 30 repetitions (15 on both legs).

4. PUSH-UPS

Push-ups are a form of workouts that will help the following parts of the body:

Shoulders or pectorals

Chest muscles or deltoids

Triceps or back of arms

Abdominals

Armpit

Benefits of Push-ups

• They are excellent for bodywork.

- They help in making the body balance and stable.
- They aid the building of muscle density.
- Push-ups help in improving the strong core.

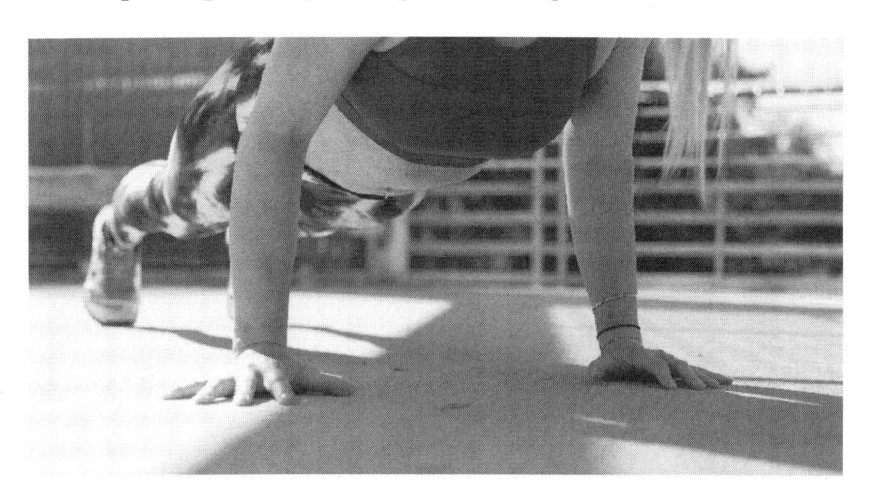

Steps:

1. Lie flat on the stomach.

2. Push body off the ground into a plank position.

3. Hold the body with toes with hands, but not forearms.

4. Low the back, there allowing the chest to touch the ground.

5. Push down palm immediately to raise the body back to a plank position.

6. Do 5 sets of 15 repetitions.

5. SIT-UPS

Sit-ups are specifically created to promote great posture for the lower back and gluteal muscles. Sit-ups will target muscles than other workouts like crunches and static core workout.

Benefits of Sit-ups

• They improve core strength.

• They help in the improvement of muscle mass.

• They will improve the performance of athletes.

• They aids balance and stability.

• Sit-ups encourage good posture.

• They are strengthening diaphragm.

• They help in the reduction of risk of back pain.

Steps:

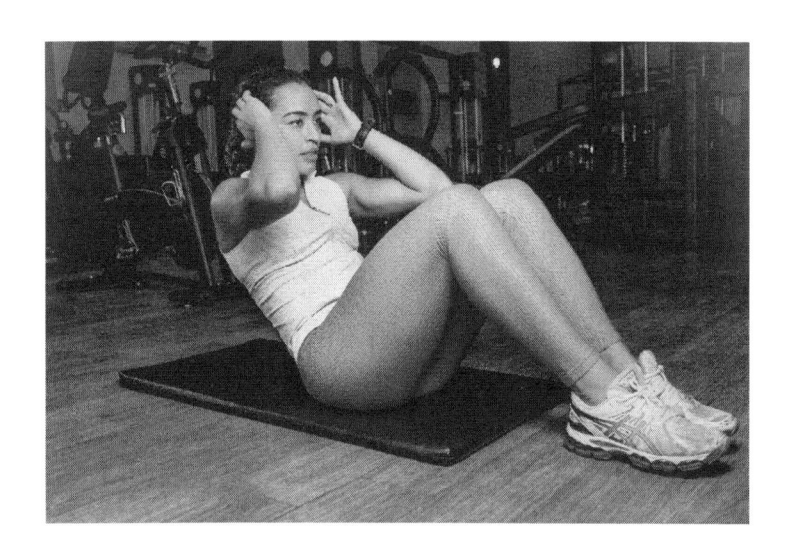

1. Lie flat on the back with legs bent and feet flat on the ground.

2. Put the hands beneath the neck with elbows out to the sides.

3. Clench the stomach muscles and bring out the torso up so to flush with thighs.

4. Don't allow the urge to use momentum, but muscles to ring the body up.

5. Protect the body down in a controlled motion to make good use of the muscle core.

6. Do the 5 sets of 25 repetitions.

6. JUMP ROPE

Jump rope is an excellent exercise as it helps in burning calorie. This workout is useful to the extent that it will help in burning 200 to 300 calories in 13 minutes.

Benefits of Jump rope

• The jump rope will help in burning calorie.

• They help in the improvement of coordination.

• Help in the reduction of injury risk.

• Aids the condition of heart health.

• The right way to strengthening bone density.

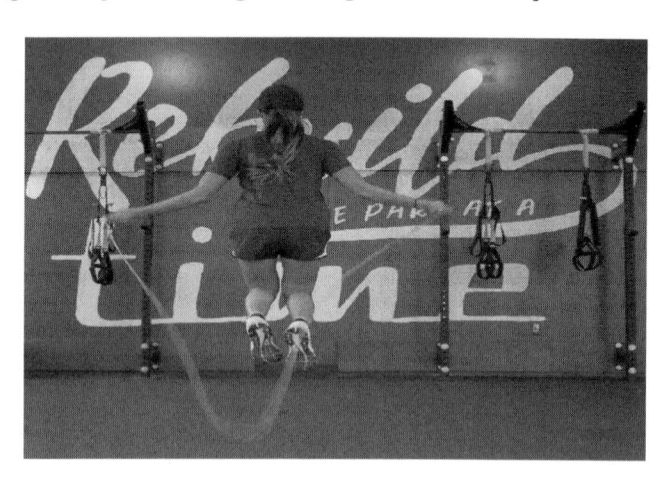

Steps:

1. Get a jump rope and a good pair of shoes.

2. Turn a rope with handles repeatedly while you jump over it.

3. To avoid accidents as a beginner, turn the rope with your wrists, not with your arms and land softly.

4. Don't jump too high to avoid an accident.

5. Do continues jumping of 10 to 30 seconds for a set.

6. Do 5 set of 10 repetitions?

7. JUMPING JACKS

Jumping jacks are great workout tools for the total body that can be done almost anywhere. They work majorly on muscle, lungs, and heart. Jumping jacks are known to burn more than 100 calories in 10 minutes. Other parts that they affect are;

Quadriceps

Glutes

Hip flexors

Shoulder muscles

Abdominals

Benefits Jumping jacks

• They help in the management of weight.

• Help to reduce blood pressure.

• Help to reduce and cholesterol.

• Help to increase insulin sensitivity in the body.

• Help to increase good cholesterol.

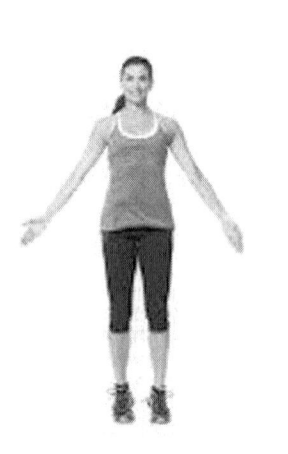

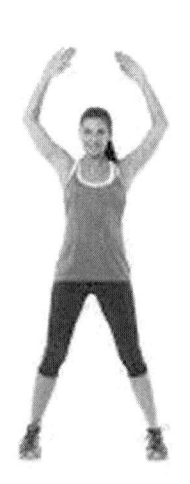

Steps:

1. Get a good pair of shoes.

2. Jump repeatedly while the feet apart and cycling the arms overhead.

3. Repeat for the next 45 to 60 seconds and stop.

4. Repeat until you can go for 2 minutes at a stretch

8. BURPEES

Burpees are kinds of workouts that will work on major muscle groups in the body. They are in two-part, push and leap in the air.

Burpees are so great in burning calories that if a person of 185 pounds can do 20 minutes, it will burn 15 calories.

Benefits of Burpees

• They work on the total body.

• They improve cardio fitness and help in burning fats.

• Burpees are versatile and convenient.

• Burpees require no special equipment.

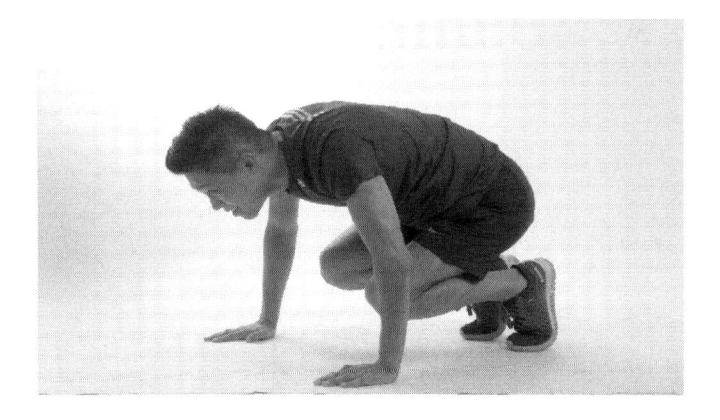

Steps:

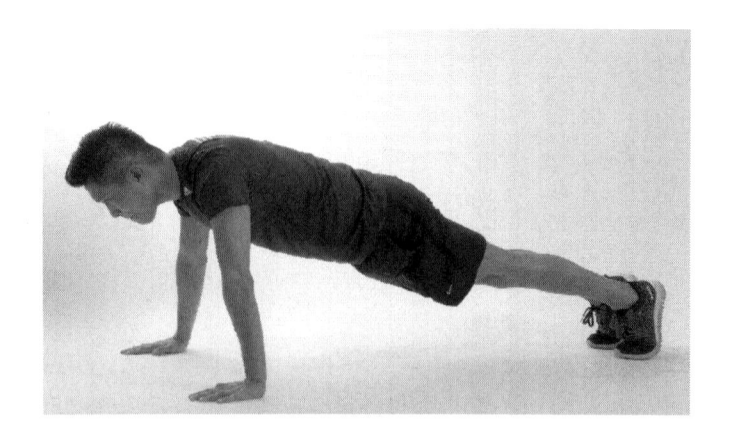

1. Squat with knees bent, back straight and feet about shoulder-width apart.

2. Low the hands to the floor in fronts o to inside the feet.

3. With the weight on the hands, kick feet back to be on hands and toes, and in a push-up state.

4. Keep the body straight from head to heels with one push-Up.

5. Don't allow the back to sag or to stick butt in the air.

6. Frog kick by jumping the feet to their former position.

7. Sit and reach the arms over the head.

8. Quickly jump into the air so to land at the former position.

9. Once landed with the knees bent, get into the squat position and repeat the steps.

10. Do 45 to 60 seconds of Burpees and rest for 45 to 60 seconds.

11. Repeat for 10 minutes or more.

9. MOUNTAIN CLIMBERS

Mountain Climbing is a kind of workout that will stretch your core and also work on muscular endurance with cardio.

Mountain climbers work on wrists, shoulders, and arms.

Benefits of Mountain Climbers

• Improve flexibility.

• Great for the butt.

• Lower body strength boosters.

• Can be done anywhere.

• Great for the heart.

• Enhanced mobility.

• Great for your balance.

- Burn fat.

- Make you stronger.

- Excellent for strengthening the core.

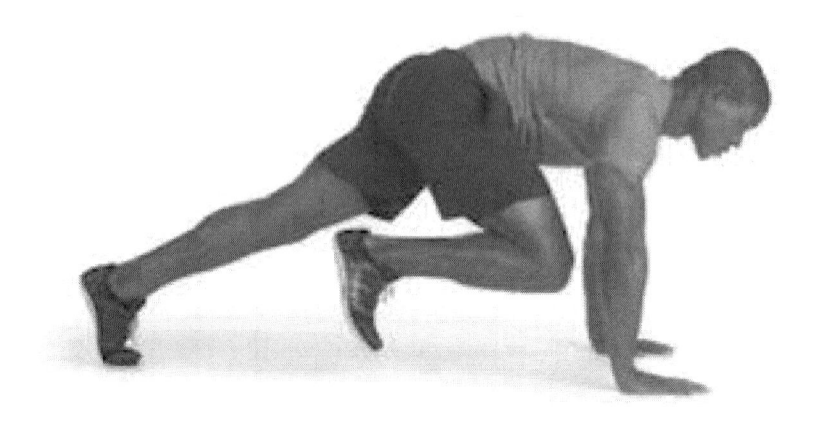

Steps:

1. Get down with both your arms and legs on the floor as a push-up.

2. Keep running the knees in and out from a push position.

3. Alternate left leg and right leg forward and backwards.

4. Do the processes between 45 to 60 seconds.

5. Repeat the cycle in 10 minutes.

10. BEAR CRAWL PUSH-UPS

This is a variation of bear crawl hold that comes with push-ups. Its major work is to add extra coordination, strengthens shoulders and help a range of muscle groups, core, and legs.

Benefits of Bear Crawl Push-ups

• Encourages Engagement

• Better Workout Efficiency

• Improves Athletic and Daily Performance

• May Boost Cognitive Functioning

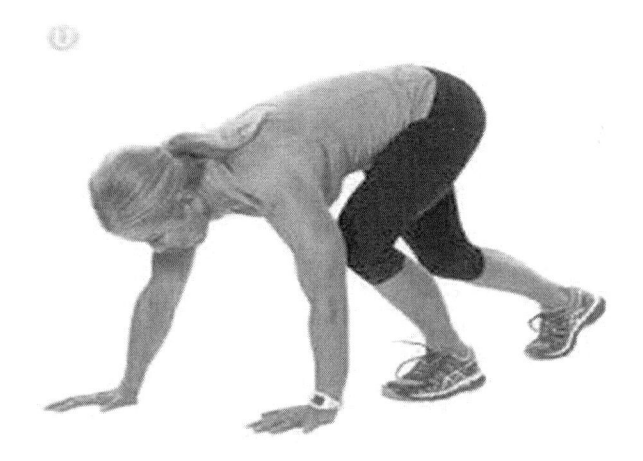

Steps:

1. Move forward by moving right hand and left leg forward in

a crawling manner.

2. Place weight on the right hand and left leg.

3. Then switch sides and move the left hand and right leg forward.

4. Keep your body low and continue with crawling movement.

5. Do this in 5 to 8 steps, and take a short break of 30 to 60 seconds.

11. STAIRCASE EXERCISE

There are reports that show that adding staircase climbing to your workout will help in strengthening and toning of leg muscles. This work out will keep leg arteries flexible, thereby allowing blood to circulate efficiently. There is a study that said that it is better to climb 10 to 12 stairs so to burn 2 to 5 calories.

Benefits of Staircase Exercise

• This burn more calories than jogging.

• Easy to do than other workouts.

- Can be used to manage weight and in building muscle tone.
- Help in reducing cardio risk.

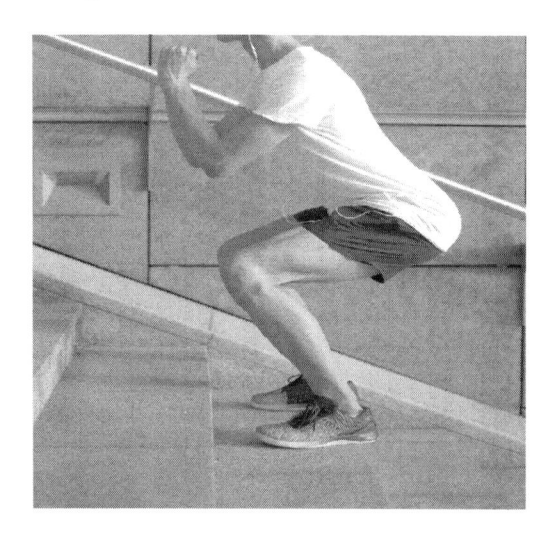

Steps:

1. Squat on the floor

2. Walk your hand to do push-ups

3. Walk the hand back and stand up.

4. Do it 45 to 60 seconds, then rest for 45 to 60 seconds.

5. Repeat the steps for 10 minutes or more.

SHOPPING LIST FOR CARB CYCLING

This is for 1 Serving

Snacks & Nuts

Walnuts	15.1 gm
Sesame seeds	18.2 gm
Cashew milk, unsweetened	20.8 ml
Pistachio nuts	8.1 gm
Pumpkin seeds	4.9 gm
Almond butter	16.2 gm
Brazil nuts	99.3 gm
Goji berries	21 gm
Sunflower seeds	9 gm
Coconut, shredded, unsweetened	39.1 gm
Cashew nuts, raw	25.8 gm
Peanut butter, natural	32.8 gm
Chia seeds	14.4 gm

Condiments

Sesame oil	11.2 ml
Tabasco sauce	2.5 ml
Vanilla extract, pure	4.9 ml
Walnut oil	22.4 ml

Coconut aminos, Coconut Secret	15.6 ml
Coconut oil	54.2 gm
Tamari, gluten free, reduced sodium	15.0 ml
Mayonnaise	9.3 gm
Olive oil	1.1 ml
Extra virgin olive oil	134.3 ml
Dijon mustard	17.1 gm
Apple cider vinegar	286.5 ml

Fruits

Apple	3.6 Medium
Raspberries	32.5 gm
Avocado	0.5 (Avocados)
Blueberries	38.3 gm
Mango	0.7

Beverage

Almond milk, unsweetened, Blue Diamond	250.0 ml
Lime juice	7.4 ml

Vegetables

White onion	0.5 Medium
Yellow onion	0.3 Medium
Zucchini	0.1 Medium
Carrots	4.4 Medium
Celery	0.8 Medium stalks
Cherry Tomatoes	6.5 Tomatoes
Garlic	0.5 gm
Ginger root	0.1 piece, 2-inch
Ginger, dried	2 gm
Artichoke heart, raw	64 gm
Baby spinach	760.8 gm
Red onion	8.3 gm
Sauerkraut	262.6 gm
Spinach	47.5 gm
Parsley, fresh	7.6 gm
Potato	2 potatoes
Basil, fresh	9.8 leaf
Green cabbage	0.2 Medium head
Kale	1.0 bunch
Beets, raw	0.5 (beets)
Butternut squash	0.5
Cremini (Italian) mushroom	2.7

Orange bell pepper	0.5
Tomato	0.3 medium
Sweet onion	0.7
Broccoli florets	0.8 bag (16 oz)
Garlic	0.5 bulb
Green onion, scallion, ramp	0.1 bunch
Green/yellow string beans, raw	39.4 gm
Lettuce, romaine	<0.1 head
Button mushrooms	0.1 (8oz)

Spices & Herbs

Nutmeg, ground	4.4 gm
Rosemary, dried	2.4 gm
Rosemary, fresh	0.3 gm
Salt	9.6 gm
Black pepper	5.1 gm
Cinnamon	7.0 gm
Ginger, ground	0.9 gm
Himalayan sea salt	1.0 gm
Salt and pepper	0.3 gm
Basil pesto	20 gm
Sea salt	4.2 gm

Turmeric, powder	1.1 gm
Thyme, fresh	<0.1 bunch

Seafood

Atlantic salmon, wild	200 gm
Atlantic salmon, farmed	113.4 gm

Meat

Bacon	45.3 gm
Turkey, deli cut	56 gm
Whole Chicken	575 gm
Chicken breast, boneless, skinless	0.8 breast
Chicken thighs, bone-in, skinless	4 thighs

Pasta & Rice

Brown rice pasta	42.5 gm

Baking

Maple syrup	9.9 ml
Vanilla bean paste	3.8 gm
Cacao powder	5.4 gm

Coconut flour	4.7 gm
Honey	50.1 gm
Honey, raw	1.2 tablespoons
Dark chocolate chips, vegan	<0.1 package

Others

Hemp protein powder	28 gm
Stevia	5.4 gm
Egg, hard boiled	1.1 medium egg
Cannellini beans, canned	0.3 can (15oz)

Canned Food

Tomato paste, canned	0.1 small can
Tomato sauce, canned	0.1 can(s) (15oz)
Coconut milk, reduced fat	500.0 ml
Olives	8.5 gm
Chicken broth (stock)	222.2 ml
Coconut milk	343.7 ml
Vegetable stock/broth	0.1 box

Dairy & Cheese

| Goat cheese, semi- | 9.4 gm |

soft	
Goat cheese, soft	9.4 gm
Egg	5.7 medium egg
Ghee	14.4 gm

Frozen & Refrigerated Foods

Frozen spinach	0.1 package (10oz)
Yoso Plain Unsweetened Coconut Yogurt	0.6 container

Cereals

Rolled oats- Gluten Free	164.8 gm

WHAT IS GLYCEMIC INDEX?

Glycemic index is a number that tells how fast the human body will convert the carbs in a food into glucose. Two different meals of the same amount carbs may have different glycemic index numbers. According to the Glycemic index, the smaller the index number, the lesser will be the impact of the food on the blood sugar.

Note that the glycemic index on its own is not a diet plan but one of the useful tools in dieting. Its main work is to help in the calorie counting or carb counting to be able to guide the choices of food. Factors that affect the glycemic index of food include the composition of food nutrient, the method by which a portion of food is cooked, and the amount of process it has undergone.

According to the glycemic index, foods are classified as low, medium, and high index as they are ranked from 0 to 100. Once again, the lesser the index number, the lower it may affect blood sugar.

Three GI ratings:

Bad: 55 or less Low

Medium: 56 to 69

Bad: 70 or higher (High)

Note: You can find the glycemic index on the labels of the packaged foods, or can be found on the internet.

List of foods that are appropriate for low diet:

Fruits: grapefruit, oranges, apples, berries, lemons, limes.

Legumes: kidney beans, black beans, lentils, chickpeas.

Whole grains: oats, quinoa, barley, couscous, buckwheat, faro.

Non-starchy vegetables: tomatoes, broccoli, carrots, cauliflower, spinach.

Herbs and spices: cinnamon, turmeric, cumin, dill, basil, black pepper, rosemary.

Seeds: flax seeds, hemp seeds, chia seeds, sesame seeds.

Meat: lamb, beef, pork, bison.

Poultry: goose, turkey, chicken, duck.

Seafood: sardines, salmon, mackerel, shrimp, anchovies, tuna.

Nuts: walnuts, macadamia nuts, almonds, pistachios.

Oils: coconut oil, olive oil, vegetable oil, avocado oil.

GLYCEMIC INDEX CHART

High-Carbohydrate Foods

White wheat bread*	75 ± 2
Whole wheat/whole meal bread	74 ± 2
Specialty grain bread	53 ± 2
Unleavened wheat bread	70 ± 5
Wheat roti	62 ± 3
Chapatti	52 ± 4
Corn tortilla	46 ± 4
White rice, boiled*	73 ± 4
Brown rice, boiled	68 ± 4
Barley	28 ± 2
Sweet corn	52 ± 5
Spaghetti, white	49 ± 2
Spaghetti, whole meal	48 ± 5
Rice noodles†	53 ± 7
Udon noodles	55 ± 7
Couscous†	65 ± 4
White wheat bread*	75 ± 2

Breakfast Cereals

Cornflakes	81 ± 6

Wheat flake biscuits	69 ± 2
Porridge, rolled oats	55 ± 2
Instant oat porridge	79 ± 3
Rice porridge/congee	78 ± 9
Millet porridge	67 ± 5
Muesli	57 ± 2

Fruit and Fruit Products

Apple, raw†	36 ± 2
Orange, raw†	43 ± 3
Banana, raw†	51 ± 3
Pineapple, raw	59 ± 8
Mango, raw†	51 ± 5
Watermelon, raw	76 ± 4
Dates, raw	42 ± 4
Peaches, canned†	43 ± 5
Strawberry jam/jelly	49 ± 3
Apple juice	41 ± 2
Orange juice	50 ± 2

Vegetables

Potato, boiled	78 ± 4
Potato, instant mash	87 ± 3

Potato, French fries	63 ± 5
Carrots, boiled	39 ± 4
Sweet potato, boiled	63 ± 6
Pumpkin, boiled	64 ± 7
Plantain/green banana	55 ± 6
Taro, boiled	53 ± 2
Vegetable soup	48 ± 5

Dairy Products and Alternatives

Milk, full fat	39 ± 3
Milk, skim	37 ± 4
Ice cream	51 ± 3
Yogurt, fruit	41 ± 2
Soy milk	34 ± 4
Rice milk	86 ± 7

Legumes

Chickpeas	28 ± 9
Kidney beans	24 ± 4
Lentils	32 ± 5
Soya beans	16 ± 1

Snack Products

Chocolate	40 ± 3
Popcorn	65 ± 5
Potato crisps	56 ± 3
Soft drink/soda	59 ± 3
Rice crackers/crisps	87 ± 2

Sugars

Fructose	15 ± 4
Sucrose	65 ± 4
Glucose	103 ± 3
Honey	61 ± 3

This chart belongs to **www.health.harvard.edu**

Chapter 4

CARB CYCLING DIET PLAN

Below is a sample menu of how your one week of carb cycling should look like.

DAY 1 MONDAY: LOW CARB DAY

A small portion of whole grains or/and a small portion of starchy veggies after exercises.

There should not be a drink after exercises.

There should be fruit.

The rest of the day should come with healthy fats, lean proteins, fibrous vegetable or greens.

DAY 2 TUESDAY: HIGHER CARB DAY

A small portion of whole grains or/and a small portion of starchy veggies

There should not be a drink after exercises.

Eat fruits.

The rest of the day should come with healthy fats, lean proteins, fibrous vegetable or greens.

DAY 3 WEDNESDAY: LOW CARB DAY

A small portion of whole grains or/and a small portion of starchy veggies after exercises.

There should not be a drink after exercises.

There should be fruit.

The rest of the day should come with healthy fats, lean proteins, fibrous vegetable or greens.

DAY 4 THURSDAY: HIGHER CARB DAY

A small portion of whole grains or/and a small portion of starchy veggies

There should not be a drink after exercises.

Eat fruits today.

The rest of the day should come with healthy fats, lean proteins, fibrous vegetable or greens.

DAY 5 FRIDAY: LOW CARB DAY

A small portion of whole grains or/and a small portion of starchy veggies after exercises.

There should not be a drink after exercises.

There should be fruit today.

The rest of the day should come with healthy fats, lean proteins, fibrous vegetable or greens.

DAY 6 SATURDAY: HIGHER CARB DAY

A small portion of whole grains or/and a small portion of starchy veggies

There should not be a drink after exercises.

Eat fruits today.

The rest of the day should come with healthy fats, lean proteins, fibrous vegetable or greens.

DAY 7 SUNDAY: MODERATE CARB DAY

A small portion of whole grains or/and a small portion of starchy veggies after exercises.

There should not be a drink after exercises.

There should be fruits.

Eat fruit today.

The rest of the day should come with healthy fats, lean proteins, fibrous vegetable or greens.

So it is expected that your week should be like this:

Day	Carb Intake	Fat Intake	Exercise	Amount of Carbs
Monday	Low carb	High fat	Aerobic Workout	< 50g
Tuesday	High carb	Low fat	Weight Training	200g
Wednesday	Low carb	High fat	Rest Day	< 50g
Thursday	High carb	Low fat	Weight Training	200g
Friday	Low carb	High fat	Aerobic Workout	< 50g
Saturday	High Carb	Low fat	Weight Training	200g

| Sunday | Moderate carb | Moderate fat | Rest Day | 100g |

The Carb cycling can be tuned and recreated to suit your purpose. You can experiment with the amount of both high carb and low carb days per week, and also the amount of carbs per day. Yours is just to know the kind of lifestyle, daily routine, and workout you engage.

COMMON MISTAKES NOT TO MAKE IN CARB CYCLING

Not knowing how long to be on a low carb diet:

No two ways to it than to dare to take some experiments with the diet. If you are a type that quickly gains weight and overweight, it will be advisable to be on a low carb diet for 5 to 6 days. However, if you are the type that possesses a higher metabolic rate and your goal is to shed a few extra pounds, what you need is a 3 to 4 days of low car alternatively with high carb days. If you discover that there are no results, just add more day to the low carb period.

Not consuming the correct amount of calories daily:

If your aim is to have a 450 to a 550 calorie daily. So it is expected that you should not go below or above this range if you are to achieve the maximum results. Note that if you go

below, fat loss will be slow. If you consume less calories, your body will enter starvation mode, and there won't be fat loss.

Consumption of wrong types of carbs:

The day meant to eat clean starchy carbs such as brown or white potatoes, brown or white rice or any other tuber, but you change your mind to change it to doughnut and cakes will truncate the results. You have to follow the guidelines religiously.

Exceeding the desired calorie intake on a high carb day:

Don't try to stuff your high day with all kinds of junk foods. Though high carb day is known to be a cheat day, so don't shoot yourself in the feet. Aim for what you are expected to consume for that day.

SAMPLE MENU

Day 1 Monday: Low Carb Day

Breakfast + Snacks

Lunch + Snacks

Dinner + Snacks

Day 2 Tuesday: Higher Carb Day

Endurance/ cardio

Breakfast + Snacks

Lunch + Snacks

Dinner + Snacks

Day 3 Wednesday:

Low Carb Day

Breakfast + Snacks

Lunch + Snacks

Dinner + Snacks

Day 4 Thursday:

Higher Carb Day

Endurance/ cardio

Breakfast + Snacks

Lunch + Snacks

Dinner + Snacks

Day 5 Friday: Low Carb Day

Breakfast + Snacks

Lunch + Snacks

Dinner + Snacks

Day 6 Saturday: Higher Carb Day

Endurance/ cardio

Breakfast + Snacks

Lunch + Snacks

Dinner + Snacks

Day 7 Sunday: Moderate Carb Day

Breakfast + Snacks

Lunch + Snacks

Dinner + Snacks

PREPPING YOUR MEALS IN EASY WAYS

We have covered what determines overweight, obesity, what foods to eat, and what not to eat. It is important to know and understand how to make your healthy high and low carb meal by yourself. It is advisable that in this journey of weight loss, it is preferable to prepare your meals ahead of time. If you want the carb cycling recipes in this book to work for you, you will have to eat the right foods at the right time.

You need to have your foods ahead of time, as it will one day safe you from the unforeseen situation. Imagine if you don't have the required foods when you are hungry? Definitely, you may need to have what is available. This will jeopardize your progress and may lead to starting again.

The main reason why you need to prep your food in bulk is to prepare for long term goal. With how busy our schedules are these days, I don't think it is reasonable to prepare a meal every three hours. So the best is to prepare your foods in bulk two times a week, preferably Sunday, and Wednesday. The one preparing should be able to last between three to four days. The rest is to know how to combine the prepared and enjoy the meals. With this in place, you don't have to be thinking of what to cook; yours is just to follow the carb cycling diet plan.

Don't be troubled. It is possible for you to prepare your food for three or four days within an hour. If you prep it in bulk, portion it immediately and keep in separate containers. Get plastic containers from the store and portion it in them, and then store in the refrigerator.

FOODS THAT ARE EASY AND ARE ON THE GO

Are you the type that doesn't have time to prep your foods due to the nature of your lifestyle? The following are some of the best foods you can quickly get:

Carbohydrates

• Majority of fruits comes naturally in portion. So get enough and keep in the kitchen. Know that some can be refrigerated while some cannot.

• Get canned lentils and beans to have carbs and protein.

• You can use whole-grain bread and tortilla for sandwiches, burritos, and wraps.

• Oatmeals can be microwaved for a couple of minutes. You can also use a blender to blend dry oatmeal with protein shakes.

• Potatoes, sweet potatoes and yams can be prepared with a microwave.

• Low-fat/low-sugar cereal and granola are high-fiber grains that can be stored.

Proteins

• Proteins such as legume powder, whey powder, soy powder and egg powder are easy and less expensive to get. They can be substituted for any other protein in your diet plan. These protein powders come in different flavors, and when some are mixed, they taste like a milkshake.

- Plain Greek yoghurt, cottage cheese and nonfat are protein on the go foods. These foods can be combined with fruits, eaten plain, sweetened with stevia, and substituted for sour cream.
- Beef, chicken, and canned fish are also good foods.
- Roast beef, sliced turkey, and chicken.

Fat

Low-fat cheese

Pecans, almonds, and walnuts

Avocados

Peanut butter

Blue cheese

Vegetables

Carrots

Cucumbers

Peppers

Celery

Mixed salads

Chapter 5

LOW CARB DAYS RECIPES

BREAKFAST

1. Breakfast: Peel 1 grapefruit and 1 orange and cut the segments into halve. Then mix the combination with yoghurt, some quantity of blueberries and 2 tablespoons of almond (crushed). Ready to be consumed.

Snack: Eat 1 Apple

2. Breakfast: Combine 2 tablespoons of rolled oats and 2 tablespoons of pumpkin seeds, sesame seeds, and sunflower seed. Soak the combination for 30 minutes in the fridge, placing in semi-skimmed milk. Add 1 small grated apple, 2 tablespoons before serving.

Snack: Some pieces of walnuts, and 1 banana.

3. Breakfast: 1/2 red pepper, 3 eggs, 1/2 onion, 2 tablespoons yoghurt, 1/2 courgette, salt, 1 tablespoon, and pepper in medium pan and cook.

Snack: 1 Apple, and large quantities of pumpkin seeds.

4. Breakfast: 2 slices of toasted wholemeal pitta spread with butter (unsalted) and marmite, 2 boiled eggs.

Snack: 1 Apple and 1 pear.

5. Breakfast: 2 large grilled tomatoes, 2 poached eggs, and 2 Portobello mushrooms.

Snack: 1 orange, 1 peach, and 150g of natural yoghurt.

6. Breakfast: Toasted and caramelized banana

Snack: 1 cup of coffee and 1 scoop of whey protein powder.

LUNCH

1. Lunch: Put 50g of grain quinoa in water and cook. Combine sliced cucumber, 100g chopped tomatoes, 2 chopped hard-boiled eggs, and 100g of garden peas.

Snack: 1 Banana, and a handful of walnuts.

2. Lunch: 1/2 Avocado, 1 wholemeal pitta bread spread with tuna, and 1 tablespoon of low-fat cottage cheese.

Snack: 1 pear.

3. Lunch: Combine 1 small can of beans with 1 salmon small can. Then add 2 handfuls of lettuce leaves, 1/2 sliced onion, 1/2 tablespoon of sugar snap peas, and garnish with cider vinegar, pepper and olive oil.

Snack: 1 Banana

4. Lunch: Mix 200g can of drained tuna and 1/2 ripe of avocado. Then season it with 1/2 juice of a lime. Serve on 1 slice tomato, 1 chopped little lettuce, 1/2 carrot (grated), sliced cucumber, and 1/2 courgette.

Snack: 1 peach, and 4 oatcakes filled with cottage cheese and cucumber.

5. Lunch: Open 1 wholemeal pitta bread and fill with peanut butter. Also, fill with cottage cheese, 1/2 slice of avocado, lettuce, sliced tomato, and sliced cucumber.

Snack: 1 Nectarine, and a handful of a combination of pumpkin and sunflower seeds.

6. Lunch: combine 4 oz grilled of chicken breast, 2 cups of mixed greens, and 1/4 avocado.

Snack: 14 cashews and 1/4 cup of 4% cottage cheese.

DINNER

1. Dinner: Stir-fry chicken breast with olive oil and add little ginger (chopped). Mix 1 sliced carrot, 1 sliced courgette, and 1/2 tray of beans (green). Then add little water, soy sauce to steam. Serve it with quinoa (70g dry weight).

Snack: 2 oatcakes.

2. Dinner: Rub olive oil on a salmon steak with black pepper. Slice lime thinly and put on top of the salmon. Grill the salmon for few minutes. Serve the grilled salmon with steamed broccoli (100g), 70g of quinoa (dry weight).

Snack: 1 Apple.

3. Dinner: Roast 1 onion (chopped), 1 courgette (chopped), 1 red pepper (chopped), garlic (chopped), chili (chopped), and cumin (chopped) for 45 minutes. Rub the turkey breast with olive oil, season with salt and pepper and grill for 20 minutes. Serve with veggies.

Snack: 1 Banana and 80g of grapes.

4. Dinner: fry little ginger (chopped), 1/2 onion (chopped) in olive oil. Then stir in 1/2 courgette (chopped), 1/2 carrot (chopped), and 1/2 red pepper (chopped). Add tomatoes (400g canned), 2 teaspoons of tomato puree, and 1 can of salmon. Simmer the mixture for 10 minutes and enjoy.

Snack: 1 nectarine.

5. Dinner: Combine cherry tomatoes (200g), 1 sliced courgette, and a handful of sugar snap peas to a pan and add water to fill the mixture. Put the salmon on top of the veggies and cover it with coriander. Allow boiling, lower the heat and allow the salmon and vegetables to cook well.

Snack: 1 Banana and 2 oatcakes.

6. Dinner: combine 3 slices of bacon, 3 oz of lean ground burger, and 1 slice of Swiss cheese.

Snack: 1 cup of steamed broccoli.

Chapter 6

HIGH CARB DAYS RECIPES

BREAKFAST:

1. Breakfast: Cook oats (60g) in water. When about to cook add frozen summer berries (200g) and mix for 5 minutes until hot. Serve the mixture with 1 tablespoon of sunflower seeds and 1 pot of yoghurt (natural).

Snack: 1 peach.

2. Breakfast: Combine 5 tablespoons of natural yoghurt, 1 sliced pear, 200g of defrosted summer berries, and 1 tablespoon of honey.

Snack: 1 tomato (chopped), and 1 wholemeal pitta spread with a low-fat cottage.

3. Breakfast: combine 1 cup of shredded of wheat cereal, 1/2 sliced of a medium banana, 1/2 cup of high-protein nonfat milk, and 1 large hard-boiled egg.

Snack: 1 almond and 1 small box of raisins.

4. Breakfast: Mix 1/2 cup of high-protein nonfat milk, 3/4 cup of dry oatmeal, 1/4 cup of mixed berries and 1 tablespoon of walnuts (chopped).

Snack: Blend 1/2 grapefruit, 1 scoop of whey protein powder, and 1 small box of raisins.

5. Breakfast: blend 1/2 medium sliced banana, 1/2 whole wheat bagel, and 1 tablespoon of peanut butter.

Snack: mix 1 cup of grapes, cheese, and popcorn.

6. Breakfast: Mix 1/2 grapefruit, 2 tablespoons of cream cheese, and 1/2 whole-wheat bagel.

Snack: 2 tablespoons of peanut butter, and 1 medium apple.

LUNCH

1. Lunch: Combine 1 baked potato spread with 1 tablespoon of hummus, sliced red pepper, 1 sliced tomato, and mixed salad leaves.

Snack: 1 Apple

2. Lunch: Combine lettuce with 5 fresh salad ingredients (chopped). Then add 1/2 large can of chickpeas to the salad and garnish with olive oil and vinegar.

Snack: sliced apple, 4 oatcakes with peanut butter.

3. Lunch: Blend 1 cup of brown rice with 1 cup of lentil soup.

Snack: Mix 2 cups of frozen fruits, 1 scoop of whey protein powder, and 1/4 cup of high-protein nonfat milk.

4. Lunch: Mix 1 cup of brown rice and 1 cup of lentil soup

Snack: 1 Slice of Ezekiel bread, 1/2 medium banana sliced, and 1 tablespoon of peanut butter.

5. Lunch: 2 slices of Ezekiel bread, 2 tablespoons of mayonnaise (olive oil), and 1 white tuna.

Snack: 1/4 cup of hummus and 1 serving of Pretzels.

6. Lunch: 1 can of white tuna, 1 serving whole-grain crackers, and 1 tablespoon of mayonnaise (olive oil).

Snack: 1/4 cup of hummus and 1 serving Pretzels.

DINNER

1. Dinner; Rub 1 large cod fillet with olive oil, and then season with ground cumin and black pepper. Grill the seasoned fish. Serve with 250g of boiled potatoes, garden peas, 100g of steamed carrots, and fresh coriander.

Snack: 2 oatcakes.

2. Dinner: Rub lightly skinless chicken breast with olive oil and grill hot: steam broccoli (chopped) and 100g of green beans. Serve with chicken and dry grain quinoa (70g).

Snack: 1 Banana.

3. Dinner: 3 oz of grilled chicken breast with 1 medium of sweet potato.

Snack: 1 cup of steamed broccoli.

4. Dinner: 1 medium potato (baked), and 3 oz grilled sirloin steak.

Snack: 1 Banana.

5. Dinner: Blend 1/4 cup of tomato sauce, 1 1/2 cups of black beans, 3 oz grilled chicken breast garnish with pepper and onions, and 2 tablespoons of salsa.

Snack: 1 cup of steamed veggies.

6. Dinner: 1/2 cup of brown rice, 1/2 cup of black beans, 2 tablespoons of salsa, and 3 oz grilled chicken breast garnished with pepper and onion.

Snack: 2 tablespoons of diced tomato, and 1/4 cup of shredded romaine lettuce.

CONCLUSION

Thank you for buying this book!

I hope you have measured your progress as you journey through this diet plan. This is not a book to read for fun, but a workbook. I expect you to track your body fat and body circumference every 2 to 3 weeks. Measuring your body will make you know how effective the recipes you are consuming, and if there are any modifications to the methods or the exercise habits.

Please be informed that there is no magic about this, and you will only have progress in transformation if you take to your diet plan. The first few weeks when you start carb cycling, you will see a lot of progress quickly, but as you become thinner, the growth will not be as evident as when you first begin. Don't be discouraged; that's how it should be.

Remember, if you follow all the guidelines in this book with proper diet and exercises, be sure that you will be adding lean muscle and you will be losing fat at the same time.

So look no further, and start using this book for the dramatic transformation of your body.

Congratulations! As you make good use of this book, you will have the rest of your life in a healthier and slimmer body.

Thanks.

Reference

https://www.health.harvard.edu/diseases-and-conditions/glycemic-index-and-glycemic-load-for-100-foods (Glycemic index for 60+ foods)

https://dlife.com/high-glycemic-index-foods-to-avoid/

https://www.oxygenmag.com/nutrition/carb-cycling-for-fat-loss

https://www.healthline.com/nutrition/carb-cycling-101#section9

Printed in Great Britain
by Amazon